Table of Contents

8. Conclusion

1. Introduction

I'm excited knowing that you have purchased my 10-day smoothie cleanse book, and I'm even more excited that you're reading it. I'm delighted to have the chance to share all that I know about being healthy and preventing disease, along with my tips and recipes for making great green smoothies, also to share with you how you can spoil your body in such an easy and tasty way.

I'm thrilled that you've chosen this book to help start you on an adventure that can take you, your body, and even your mind and emotions to places you never thought you'd go. And I'm glad to be part of the spark that guides you toward drinking your way to better health.

I have been drinking smoothies my entire life and am a firm believer in the amazing weight loss and health benefits they possess. A high quality smoothie allows you to blend lots of nutrient dense ingredients into one drink. I like to think of a smoothie as a one stop shop for optimal health and fitness.

The following smoothie recipes are geared towards boosting your energy levels, metabolism and fat burning potential. These smoothies also contain some of the highest antioxidant foods in the world.

When you are looking to boost your overall health and lose weight you need proper nutrition. These smoothies are high in every essential vitamin and mineral and many contain "green" ingredients such as Spinach and Kale. These green ingredients should not intimidate you – and in fact mix deliciously with tropical fruit. Kale is one of the most nutrient dense foods in the world and is a great way to boost your immune system and fat burning potential.

Delicious Go for it!

2. Getting Started

To create a green smoothie you do not need much ingredients or equipment's. A few basic materials are all you need and you can start.

1: A blender:

For the making of the recipe, so you can use any blender that there is on the market. It is advisable for you to purchase a blender with a capacity of at least a half-gallon so you can prepare an entire recipe in a blender at one time If the volume of your blender is less than you may choose to add Ingredients in small steps With a little patience every blender can handle the recipes.

2: Knives

Having a good knife is half the battle won. For the recipes you need a lot of fruit and vegetable carving. A good sharp knife with a strong handle will ensures that slice your fruits and vegetables quickly and efficiently.

3: Sieve

Washing your fruits and vegetables is very important and a handy screen helps you with this. Personally, I find a screen that you can hang over the sink very convenient. You have here both hands free to properly wash your vegetables

4: Fruit and vegetables

The best option for your body is for you to use organic fruits and vegetables, but this is unfortunately not always feasible. If you use non-organic ingredients, always make sure that you give them extra good wash before use.

5: Glass jars

The great thing about green smoothies is that you can make them in advance and then refrigerate for up to two days. The best way to keep your smoothie is in a glass jar because glass is an inert substance and emits no toxic substances in your smoothie like plastic does.

3. All You Need To Know About Cleanse

What is a Cleanse?

Cleansing is the detoxification of the digestive track, blood, intestines, kidneys, liver, and lungs.

Why is cleansing important?

The evolution of modern society has resulted in an overload of chemicals, toxins, air pollutants, and radiation. In addition, by eating certain foods, we expose ourselves to processed and demineralized materials, herbicides, pesticides, food colorings, and preservatives.

The presence of these toxins put stress on our bodies. When the body is clean and strong, it has no trouble eliminating the waste. However, when it becomes overloaded with more toxins than it can properly eliminate, the liver will eventually become sluggish and allow the waste to build up. In this state, one cannot properly absorb vitamins, nutrients, and health supplements.

Also, the resulting contamination and malnutrition makes the body more susceptible to disease. In fact, a continuous overload of toxins into the body could trigger serious ailments, and if a system becomes so contaminated that it cannot get rid of the excess toxins, chronic illness or even death could result.

Difference between a Detox and a Cleanse

Detox: If you want to eliminate all of the toxins from your system, you do a detox. The goal is to eliminate heavy metals, cigarette toxins, and environmental toxins that you come into contact with via touch or breathing, chemicals that you may absorb from cleaning agents or chemicals, and just about any other foreign, toxic substance that may be floating around in your bloodstream just waiting to make you sick. Since your main goal here is healing, you may want to use juice to detox because it makes digestion simple; your digestive tract doesn't have to extract the nutrients from fiber, and the energy saved can be used for healing.

Cleanse: If you want to clean out your digestive tract from top to bottom of all toxins, parasites, lingering fecal matter, or fungi such as candida, then you'll want to do a cleanse. Smoothies are great for cleansing because the fiber in the produce sweeps all of this junk right out of your system, while the phyto-nutrients and antioxidants in the plants work to heal you and fight disease and free radicals that cause sickness and aging.

Advantages of Doing a Smoothie Cleanse

So what are the advantages of doing a smoothie cleanse versus a juice fast or detox? There are several, but which one is better for you depends entirely upon your personal health and your goals. The primary difference is that since you are still eating fiber, your body isn't getting the mad rush of nutrients that can initially cause nausea, vomiting, and headaches in people new to juicing.

Should you be cleansing?

If you are considering whether you should go do a cleanse or not, the following is a guide for you to consider.

• You have been working very hard or been under a lot of stress.

• You eat sugar or white flour and/or drink a lot of caffeine or alcohol.

• Your eyes are not clear and/or they are yellowish or red.

• You took a pH test and tested acidic.

• You feel a cold or flu coming on.

• You feel congested from too much food or the wrong kinds of food.

• You feel lethargic, like you need a good spring cleaning.

• You need to eliminate drug residues, or normalize after an illness or a hospital stay.

• You need a jump start for a healing program.

• You need a specific detox program for a serious health problem.

• You want to streamline your body processes for more energy.

• You need to remove toxins that are causing a health problem.

• You want to prevent disease and/or rest and rejuvenate the whole body.

• You want to assist with weight Joss and/or want to clear up your skin.

• You want to slow aging and improve body flexibility.

• You want to improve fertility.

• You want greater mental clarity.

- You need better quality of sleep.

- You desire freedom from negative thoughts and feelings.

- You need to improve your circulation.

How Do You Prepare for Your Cleanse

A smoothie cleanse isn't quite as traumatic to your system as a juice detox because you are still consuming fiber; even so, you'll want to prepare your body for the change in order to lessen or avoid the side effects. Here are a few tips that will help make your transition to a smoothie-only diet a little bit easier.

- Stop smoking two weeks before your cleanse.

- Eliminate dairy, simple sugars, caffeine, and processed foods three days prior to cleansing.

- Add more large, leafy salads and fresh fruit three days prior to your cleanse.

- Stock up on organic fruits and vegetables the day before you start.

- Increase your water intake to give your body a jump-start on flushing out toxins.

- Be positive about your upcoming cleanse—think of it as a gift to yourself!

- Determine how long you're going to cleanse. Typically, three to five days is sufficient.

Now you know what measures you can take to make your cleanse as simple and painless as possible, but it's true there will still be some side effects, both good and bad, that you should expect once you start. Remember, these are perfectly normal, so stick with it! If you cheat even a little bit, you're defeating the purpose of the cleanse and wasting your time and hard work.

How often should I cleanse?

Optimally, on a quarterly basis or at least once per year.

How long should I cleanse?

Cleanses last anywhere from 24 hours to 10 days. A 24-hour cleanse is a good way to deter oncoming cold and/or flu symptoms. A general cleanse lasts 3-7 days. It removes excess amounts of mucous, old fecal matter, trapped cellular and non-food wastes, and inorganic mineral deposits that contribute to arthritis. It also purifies your liver, kidneys, and blood; enhances mental clarity; increases energy; relieves the body of dependency on habit-forming substances; and reduces your stomach to its normal size contributing to weight loss.

Finally, a deep cleanse lasts for up to 10 days and can help to fight a chronic illness or disease.

In the pages to come, you'll find guidelines for 10 Days cleanse schedule, as well as a collection of favorite recipes to get you started. Remember that if you cheat or give up, the only person that you're shorting is yourself. Think positive, picture yourself healthy, and then jump in with both feet — you won't regret it

4. What to Expect During Your 10-Day Cleanse

In the first few days of your cleanse, you may feel worse before you feel better. This is because every cell in your body is dumping the toxic residue that it has absorbed from the air you breathe, the food you eat, and the environment you live in. You may experience mood swings or general crankiness as emotional debris is cleared out along with food debris. If you experience these discomforts, try to think of them as "growing pains"— they are indicators of the growing spaciousness inside you that will result in a remarkable transformation. These "growing pains" will recede as you continue the cleanse.

Allow your body to cleanse, clear, and go through the cleanup it needs. Observe what your body is telling you as you move through the 10 days of your cleanse. Know that the journey is well worth any rough spots you may encounter along your path.

Common "cleansing events" may occur at any given time during your cleanse. Continue to drink lots of pure filtered water and teas to keep flushing them out. Remember, you may experience one or two of these "events," or you may experience none at all. And no two cleanses will result in the same exact detox events. Below is a likely scenario of what you may go through during your 10 days cleans

Day One

What you may be feeling:

You may feel tired during the day and you will probably experience hunger pains.

Day Two

What you may be feeling:

Again, you may feel tired during the day and you will probably experience hunger pains, nausea, weakness, and vomiting. Also you may become irritable, have a foggy brain, be somewhat sweaty (the skin is an avenue of elimination), and have a unique body pungency. All of these are normal reactions as the toxins begin to move through your body.

Day 3

What you may be feeling:

Again, you may feel tired during the day and you will probably experience hunger pains. In addition, you may experience nausea and weakness. You may become irritable, have a foggy brain, be somewhat sweaty (the skin is an avenue of elimination), and have a unique body pungency. Also, you may get the shakes, feel out of control, have skin eruptions, and be highly sensitive to nerve pain. All of these are normal reactions as the toxins begin to move through your body.

Day 4

What you may be feeling:

Again, you may feel tired during the day. The hunger pains will have probably passed. You may still experience nausea and weakness. You may still feel irritable, have a foggy brain, be somewhat sweaty (the skin is an avenue of elimination), and have a unique body pungency. Again, you may get the shakes, feel out of control, have skin eruptions, and be highly sensitive to nerve pain. Today, you may also get hot or cold flashes and have an acidic taste in your mouth. All of these are normal reactions as the toxins begin to move through your body.

Day 5

What you may be feeling:

You may still experience weakness. You may still feel irritable and have a foggy brain. Again, you may feel out of control, have skin eruptions, and be highly sensitive to nerve pain. You may also still have an acidic taste in your mouth and have a unique body pungency. All of these are normal reactions as the toxins begin to move through your body.

Today, you may also start to feel euphoric, feel vibrant, and feel emotionally alive.

Day 6

What you may be feeling:

You may still have a unique body pungency and you may experience gas. All of these are normal reactions as the toxins begin to move through your body. Today, you may feel euphoric, feel vibrant, and feel emotionally alive. You may also have total mental clarity, have super heightened senses, and have a sense of love and connection.

More Positive things you are likely to feel Day 7 Onward

- Exuberance
- Energy
- Deep and restoring sleep
- A feeling of lightness
- sharpened senses, particularly those of taste and smell
- A feeling of comfort "in your own skin"
- Radiant, super soft skin
- clear eyes and improved vision
- Lucid dreams
- Mental clarity
- Sexual receptiveness (yes, this does happen!)

5. How to Cope With Some of the Discomfort You Will Experience During Your Cleanse

Even if you are one of the people who experience some of the less pleasant cleansing events, there are many things you can do to assist yourself as you move through them. Different sensations are linked to different areas of your body, and as each organ dumps its toxins and begins the renewal process, different symptoms may manifest themselves. Listed below are the major organs of the body that participates in the cleanse and the symptoms each creates in your body

Your Lungs

As your lungs welcome in new breath, they may discharge old toxic emotions and the cellular damage of pollution by triggering excess mucous production. You may also experience a sense of grief, or waves of sadness. To counter these symptoms, take walks in fresh air, enjoy a soothing sauna, and fill your lungs with laughter by watching funny movies or reading funny books and comics.

Kidneys

Overworked kidneys (which can be caused by too much diet soda, stimulating caffeine, and stress, among other things) may signal the release of toxins with more frequent urination, darker or lighter urine than usual, low backache, and a feeling of general anxiety. To counter these symptoms, continue to drink water and tea, promote the free exchange of fluids by exercising lightly.

Liver

One of the most important filters in our bodies, the liver may signal cleansing events via nausea, bodily chills, episodes of sweating, and emotional releases of anger and blame. To soothe these discomforts, drink extra lemon water, walk in fresh air.

Skin

Our body's largest filtering organ, the skin is the last barrier between internal debris and total release. As you cleanse you may experience body odor; unusual breakouts; rashes; patches of dry, scaly skin; or increased sweating. Immersion in water is critical for both the internal and external body. Dry brushing turns over dead skin cells and reveals radiant new growth. Avoid all deodorants, perfumes, and commercial lotions, as these will only add to your toxic input rather than allow for the toxic release.

Olive oil is also a good alternative as a moisturizer.

Colon

As toxins are released from your colon (the organ that stores and processes waste), you may experience physical and emotional sensations that are particularly challenging. Headache, nausea, gas and bloating, and bad breath are some of the physical cleansing events associated with the colon. Emotionally, you may experience fear or anxiety concerning issues related to survival (money, security, attachment to things). To counteract these discomforts, undergoing a colon cleanse or an enema on the second day of your cleanse. After a colon cleanse or enema, make sure you get plenty of fresh air, you may also wish to have a massage that concentrates on your belly.

Lymphatic System

Lymph is a fluid that moves through the entire body, cleaning, filtering, and transporting immune cells and other important structures. To imagine how busy the lymphatic system is during your cleansing time, think of it as a busy highway shuttling away all the toxins that your body has accumulated and held onto up until now. As the lymphatic system cleans your body, the entire body responds. You may feel achy or suffer from stiff muscles, and you may develop circles under your eyes. Increasing lymph circulation will speed the cleansing process. Dry skin brushing, fresh air, light exercise, and massage all helps in achieving a healthy lymphatic circulation.

Mucous Membranes

All of our body passages that communicate with the air are lined with mucous membranes, the moist membranes that cover, protect, secrete, and absorb. As they are cleansed, you may experience a coated tongue, sinus drainage, and increased mucous in your nose or lungs. You can use a tongue scraper or spoon to keep your mouth fresh.

Drink plenty of water and detoxifying ginger tea. Fresh air and exercise, as well as breathing exercises will also work to revitalize this important line of defense against toxins in your environment.

6. Your 10 Day Green Smoothies Cleanse Plan

Smoothies are a great way to add nutrition to your diet or clean out your digestive tract so that your entire body can function optimally. The Green Smoothie Cleanse is a ten-day detox/cleanse made up of green leafy veggies, fruit, and water. Green smoothies are filling and healthy, and you will enjoy drinking them.

To keep your green "meals" interesting and varied, include a combination of both sweet and savory. It's also a good idea to use a wide variety of produce to be sure you are consuming all of the nutrients your body needs. Otherwise, you may as well just reach for that cheeseburger!

Also, each leaf vegetable contains a very small percentage of toxic substances (which is different for each vegetable) that the plant has to protect themselves. This is no problem for us because our body can detoxify these substances provided you regularly alternating vegetables. So rotate with leafy greens that you use in your smoothies. This will give your body every day to connect with other substances and cannot overloading your detoxification system occur. Take for example a smoothie with spinach Monday, Tuesday with lettuce, kale Wednesday, Thursday with chard, etc.

7. Green Smoothie Recipes

7.1. King Celery Smoothie

Requirements:

• 2 large stalks celery with leaves it (if organic) or 3 stems without leaves (if not organic) cut into pieces

• 1 apple

• 1 pear

• 1 banana

• Water as needed

Preparation:

Put the fruit in the blender and add water to the same height as the fruit and blend to a smooth consistency.

Add the celery and blend again. If necessary, add more water.

Fact!

Celery contains a large amount of fibers that do not change while they are in your intestines. These fibers helps in cleaning your colon and eliminating harmful substances. This Fibers also give you a sense of being full feeling so you will have less tendency to grab snack during the day

7.2. Red Summer Smoothie

Requirements:

- 1 ½ cup strawberries

- 1 large piece of watermelon

- Possibly a pomegranate

- 1 tablespoon lemon juice

- 1 head of lettuce of your choice

- Water as needed

Preparation:

Put the fruit in the blender and add water to 2/3 height of the fruit and blend to a smooth consistency.

Add the lettuce and blend again. If necessary, add more water.

Fact!

A pomegranate a red fruit that is about as big as an orange. Many people know this fruit mainly as an ornamental fruit during Christmas but have never eaten it them self. The fruit is the size of a large orange, obscurely six-sided, with a smooth, leathery skin that ranges from brownish yellow to red; within, it is divided into several chambers containing many thin, transparent vesicles of reddish, juicy pulp, each surrounding an angular, elongated seed. The fruit is eaten fresh, and the juice is the source of grenadine syrup, used in flavorings and liqueurs.

Pomegranates is among many antioxidant-rich foods and drinks shown to prevent disease in 1999. Antioxidants prevent the damage done to cells by free radicals, molecules that are released during the normal metabolic process of oxidation. Oxidation can lead to cancerous changes, accelerate the aging process, and contribute to heart disease and degenerative diseases such as arthritis. The antioxidants, which do occur in as many as 3 times the pomegranate in red wine, protect you from free radicals and atherosclerosis (thickening of a vein), and reduce the risk of heart disease, cancer and Alzheimer's.

7.3. Popeye peach Smoothie

Requirements:

• 2 peaches

• 1 ½ cup orange juice

• 100g chard

• 100 grams of spinach

• Water as needed

Preparation:

Stop the fruit and orange juice in the blender and blend to a smooth consistency. Then add the vegetables and blend again. If necessary, add more water.

7.4. Easy Summer Smoothie

Requirements:

- ½ head of lettuce of your choice
- 500 grams of frozen tropical fruit mix.
- Water as needed

Preparation:

Blend the lettuce with a little water until smooth. Add the fruit mixture and blend the mixture with the pulse button (if you have that feature on your blender). Then blend with the normal button all until smooth. If you do not have a pulse button, it is a wise idea to first allow things to thaw before you put it in the blender so that your blender is not overloaded. If necessary, add more water.

7.5. Green fig Smoothie

Requirements:

- 3 dried figs
- 2 pears
- Juice of ½ lemon
- 1 stalk celery
- 2 kale leaves, stems removed.
- Water as needed

Preparation:

Place the fruit and lemon juice in the blender and add water to the height of the fruit and blend to a smooth consistency.

Add the cabbage and celery and blend again. If necessary, add more water.

7.6. Pineapple Lavender smoothie

Requirements:

- 100 grams of sea lavender
- 300 grams of frozen or fresh pineapple
- Water as needed

Preparation:

Put the pineapple in the blender and add water to the height of the fruit and blend to a smooth consistency.

Add the sea lavender and blend again. If necessary, add more water.

7.7. Blueberry feisty Smoothie

Requirements:

• 1 banana

• 150 grams of blueberries

• 150 grams of spinach

• Water as needed

Preparation:

Put the fruit in the blender and add water to the height of the fruit and blend to a smooth consistency.

Add the spinach and blend again. If necessary, add more water.

7.8. Flax n berry Smoothie

Requirements:

• 2 mangoes

• 150 grams of strawberry

• 150 g chard

• Water as needed

• 1 tablespoon ground flaxseed

Preparation:

Put the fruit in the blender and add water to the height of the fruit and blend to a smooth consistency.

Add the chard and ground flaxseed and blend again. If necessary, add more water.

7.9. Pineapple Explosion

Requirements:

• 1 pineapple cut

• 1 apple

• 200 grams of spinach or lettuce of your choice (no iceberg)

• Water as needed

Preparation:

Put the fruit in the blender and add water to 2/3 height of the fruit and blend to a smooth consistency.

Add the spinach or lettuce and blend again. If necessary, add more water.

Fact:

You know that a pineapple is ripe by smelling at the bottom. If it smells sweet pineapple fruit is ripe. You can also pick at the top of the pineapple. If you easily can pull a leaf it is ripe.

7.10. Green Cleanser Smoothie

Requirements:

- 1 bunch of dandelion leaves
- ½ head of lettuce of your choice
- 2 oranges
- 1 mango
- 2 prunes
- Water as needed

Preparation:

Put the fruit in the blender and add water to the same height as the fruit and blend to a smooth consistency.

Add the dandelion and lettuce and blend again. If necessary, add more water.

Fact!

Dandelion is rich in vitamins A, B, C, D, magnesium, calcium, beta-carotene and iron and therefore this plant can help with anemia caused by low levels of iron in your body properly.

7.11. Raspy Smoothie

Requirements:

- 150 grams of raspberries

- 2 apples

- 150 grams of nettle tops

- Water as needed

Preparation:

Put the fruit in the blender and add water to the height of the fruit and blend to a smooth consistency.

Add the nettles and blend again. If necessary, add more water.

7.12. Pawpaw Smoothie

Requirements:

- 1 papaya
- 2 oranges
- Dates needed
- 200 g chard
- Water as needed

Preparation:

Put the fruit in the blender and add water to the same height as the fruit and blend to a smooth consistency.

Add the chard and blend again. If necessary, add more water.

7.13. Avocado Basil Smoothie

Requirements:

- 1 tomato
- 1 bell pepper
- 1 avocado
- 2 handfuls of spinach
- 2 stalks celery
- 1 hand fresh basil
- Water as needed
- 1 tbsp. lemon juice
- 2 apples

Preparation:

Blend the spinach and water until smooth and use the stalks celery to join stir until they themselves eventually be blended. Add the remaining ingredients and blend again until smooth. If necessary, add more water.

7.14. Goji green Smoothie

Requirements:

- 100 grams of strawberries

- 1 banana

- ½ handful of goji berries

- 3 kale leaves without stem

- Water as needed

Preparation:

Put the fruits and goji berries in the blender and add water to the height of the fruit and blend until smooth and you hear ticking sound. And you can no longer see Goji berries against the wall of the blender

Add the kale and blend again. If necessary, add more water.

7.15. Parsley citrus Smoothie

Requirements:

• 2 oranges

• ½ bunch curly parsley

• 1 large medjool date or two smaller

• Water as needed

Preparation:

Stop the fruit and date in the blender and add water to the height of the fruit and blend to a smooth consistency.

Add the parsley and blend again. Parsley is more difficult to obtain than for example spinach. You can solve this by turning the blender on longer. If necessary, add more water.

7.16. Orange top Smoothie

Requirements:

- 200 ml orange juice
- 50 grams of strawberry
- 2 bananas
- 200 grams of endive
- Water as needed

Preparation:

Put the fruit along with the orange juice in the blender and blend to a smooth consistency.

Add the endive and blend again.

You can add more water as needed to make the whole smoothie thinner.

7.17. Green mango Smoothie

Requirements:

• 1 bunch of parsley

• 2 mangoes

• Water as needed

Preparations:

Put the fruit in the blender and add water to the height of the fruit and blend to an even consistency.

Then add the parsley and blend again. If necessary, add more water.

7.18. Jammie green Smoothie

Requirements:

• ½ apple

• 2 bananas

• 1 kiwi

• 150 grams of young leaf lettuce

• 50 grams of spinach

• Water as needed

Preparations:

Put the fruit in the blender and add water to the height of the fruit and blend to a smooth consistency.

Then add the vegetables and blend again. If necessary, add more water.

7.19. Warming pineapple-ginger smoothie

Requirements:

- ½ head romaine lettuce or leaf lettuce
- 1 cup pineapple
- 1 large mango
- 1 cm ginger pressed through a garlic press
- Water as needed

Preparation:

Put the fruit and crushed ginger in the blender and add water to the same height as the fruit and blend to a smooth consistency.

Add the lettuce and blend again. If necessary, add more water.

7.20. Strawberry-Pear-Cucumber Smoothie

Requirements:

Peeled cucumber

3 - 4 pears, cut up

2 kiwis, peeled

4 strawberries

½ cup fresh mint, trimmed

Water

A teaspoon agave

Preparation:

Put all the ingredients in a blender, add a cup of water and blend and until smooth

7.21. Fresh up Smoothie

Requirements:

- 10 cm cucumber
- Juice of 1 lemon
- 1 liter of water.

Preparations:

Add all the ingredients at once to the blender and blend until smooth.

7.22. Sweet Smoothies

Requirements:

- 2 ripe bananas
- 1 ripe pear
- 1 cup grapes
- 1 head of lettuce
- Water as needed

Preparation:

Blend the grapes with water.

Now add the banana and pear with it and blend.

Finally, add the lettuce there, and blend again. If necessary, add more water.

7.23. Greeny Red Smoothie

Requirements:

2 cups red leaf lettuce, packed

2 nectarines

8 strawberries

Water

Preparation:

Put the fruits in the blender add water to the level of the fruits and blend until smooth

Add red leaf lettuce, blend until consistently smooth. If necessary add more water.

7.24. Energy Booster Smoothie

Requirements:

- 1 banana
- 1 apple
- 7 prunes
- 150 grams of spinach
- Water as needed

Preparations:

Put the fruit in the blender and add water to the same height as the fruit and blend to a smooth consistency.

Add the spinach and blend again.

If necessary, add more water.

7.25. Wheaties banana Smoothie

Requirements:

2 cups fresh-cut wheatgrass

1 mango

2 bananas

Water

Preparation:

Put the fruits in the blender (diced mango and banana) and blend until smooth.

Add the wheat grass, blend and add water progressively until smooth.

7.26. Elixir Smoothie

Requirements:

4 cups knotweed

5 - 6 young grape leaves

2 medium mangoes

Water

Preparation:

Put the diced mangoes in the blender and blend. Add the grape leaves and blend until smooth.

Gradually add the knotweed into the mixture and blend. As necessary add water

7.27. Wake Up Green Smoothie

Requirements:

A cup of spinach

A stalk celery

1 chunk of cucumber

1 frozen banana

1 cup of raspberries

½-1 avocado

1 cup of cantaloupe melon chunks

1-2 cups of water

Preparations:

Put the fruits in the blender and blend until smooth. Add the leafy greens one after the other, blend and add water until smooth.

7.28. Watermelon Green Smoothie

Requirements:

2-3 cups of watermelon

1 orange

½ banana

2 kale leave s or some dandelion leaves

A squeeze of lemon or lime

1 cup of water

Preparation:

Cut up the orange and put it with others in the blender and blend until smooth.

7.29. Apple & Melon Smoothie

Requirements:

2 cups of honeydew melon, cut into pieces

1 apple

2 tbsp. of organic live yogurt (Greek yogurt is nice and thick)

1 tbsp. lime juice

1 cup of water

Ice cubes

Preparation:

Put all the ingredients in the blender add water and blend until smooth.

Put Ice cubes and enjoy!

7.30. Green Goodness Smoothie

Requirements:

2 bananas

Royal Gala apple (1)

Bosc pear (Diced) (1)

1 cup kale

¼ cup water

Preparation:

Put all the items in a blender and blend until smooth.

8. Conclusion

Notwithstanding whether you're simply looking to add more fruits and vegetables to your daily regimen, or would like to address particular health conditions, smoothies are a great addition to your diet. If you hate the taste of vegetables but love pineapple, strawberries, and other fruits, smoothies are a terrific way to boost your vegetable intake without having to plug your nose as they go down. In a nutshell, no matter what your health goal is, smoothies can help you reach it.

You should now have several important points in hand to help make your smoothie-making adventure successful. Here's a review of a few guidelines, and perhaps a couple of new ones.

• If your smoothie tastes too strongly of vegetables, add in a cucumber, an apple, or some water.

• If your smoothie is too sweet, add a cucumber.

• Don't make more than you'll drink in a day, because fruits and vegetables begin to lose nutritional value soon after the skin is broken.

• Feel free to experiment with different flavors. If things get off track, see the first two tips.

• Remove the seeds and pits of apples, plums, and other fruits. Some of them contain toxins, while others simply taste bitter.

• You can control the spiciness of peppers by removing the seeds.

• Engage a buddy to start your journey with you—it's always easier to succeed when you have a support system!

Remember that adding smoothies to your diet isn't actually a diet; it's a healthful habit you're adding to your lifestyle as a long-term way of staying healthy, looking great, and improving your quality of life. With that in mind, find combinations of produce you truly enjoy so that you look forward to your smoothie. If it's a positive experience, it will turn into a habit that you anticipate and want to repeat!

Now that you're armed with some basic knowledge, tips, and recipes, good luck on your path to better health with delicious smoothies.

9 798746 290946